Nurse's Guide

To Graduate

School

by Brittany Stone MSN, RN

Note: The topics addressed in this guide are ideas and suggestions that the author has taken from her experience to provide guidance when applying to graduate school. They're topics to think about when approaching graduate school and do not guarantee admission into graduate school.

About the Author

Brittany has been a registered nurse for 5+ years and has recently graduated from an Adult-Gerontology-Acute Care Nurse Practitioner program. Due to her previous experiences with the graduate school process, she has become very familiar with the details and expectations that graduate schools look for in candidates. Although they were draining and negative experiences at the time, she has turned her experiences into positives, and now shares what she has learned with colleagues and friends. She currently runs the blog #Nurselyfe where she likes to blend her knowledge of graduate school, nursing and healthy living, to help nurses keep their sanity and care for themselves while caring for others.

Acknowledgements

I would like to thank my friend Vanessa for pushing me to step outside my comfort zone to originally create #Nurselyfe. Had she not inspired me to do so, this guide would have never come about.

I would like to thank my family for supporting me throughout the graduate school process, which allowed me to become great student, mother and wife.

I would like to thank my husband for being so patient with me over the years and supporting me in following my passion.

Table of Contents

Introduction

Hi, my name is Brittany, I currently run the nursing blog #Nurselyfe and am a recent Grad from an Adult Gerontology-Acute Care Nurse Practitioner program. A little bit about my story, I graduated from nursing school in 2011 and immediately started working in a Cardiac Intensive Care Unit (CICU/ICU). I gained experience with Cardiothoracic surgery patients, Cardiology patients, Ear Neck and Throat patients, Urology patients, and some Medicine ICU overflow patients. As I started my career I knew that I wanted to go back to school to get my advanced practice degree, but I wasn't sure what in. So after I got a year under my belt I applied to a program and managed to get an interview, but was rejected. This crushed me. I was upset but realized that I may need to have more experience to be considered as a competitive candidate. So I worked another year, gained some more experience, stepped into some leadership roles and applied again. This time I applied to the previous school, but others too.

Again, I received interviews for all of them and felt pretty good about them. At this time I was thinking, "this could be my year, I will finally be able to start..." well, I was rejected AGAIN! Crushed the second time! This time it really hit me hard. I thought that perhaps for the first time in my life, I would not obtain the goals I set forth for myself. To me, going to graduate school was a way to continue nursing and providing care to my patients, but without the labor-intensive aspect that bedside nursing entails. Every year that I applied and didn't get in pushed back life plans, which was very aggravating!

A couple weeks after I got the notice that I didn't get in, my husband and I had a talk and he reminded me that if this was something I truly wanted to do, I would have to go balls to the wall and fight for it. Do anything and everything I could to make myself a competitive candidate. So I obtained certifications and continued to take the challenging patients so that when the next opportunity to apply came around, I was ready. I again, applied to the same schools as previously mentioned and obtained an interview with one of the schools nearby. A week before the interview, I found out that I was pregnant (not the best timing). I was thinking about canceling all interviews and just taking myself out of the running (thinking that the next year would be the year) but my family convinced me to interview anyway and if I got in, they would help out with the baby. Well, of course you can guess, I GOT IN! I was shocked, excited, terrified and nervous. Grad school and pregnant!

Grad school has been tough, but definitely worth it! I guess the moral to my story is just because you may not get in the first time, DO NOT GIVE UP! Everything happens at the right time, just be patient and resilient. Every year I applied, and although I was rejected, I contacted the schools to see what was wrong with my application and was able to gain more information and insight in regards to what graduate programs looked for. Those years of rejection helped me create this guide for you, so I hope this guide provides you with a clearer path to graduate school. Enjoy!

The Decision to go Back

So you've decided that you want to go back to school, but you don't know where to start. First, you should probably do is ask yourself these five questions.

Why do you want to go back to school?

For more money? More responsibility? More knowledge? These are very important things that you need to figure out and know because they can have an effect how well you do and your motivation throughout it all. I personally decided to go back to school because I wanted to know more and I wanted more responsibility as well and honestly, I did want to make a little bit more money. Also, the life of a bedtime nurse is pretty physically laborious. A lot of the times I found myself getting patients out of bed that were three times my size, and it started to take a toll on my back. I soon realized that this was something that I would not be able to maintain for another 30 years, so I decided to go back to school.

What kind of student are you?

This is important to assess because it's going to effect what types of programs you search for and whether or not you will be successful in the program you choose. Are you somebody who likes to work alone and go at your own pace, or are you somebody who likes to be physically in class, working with classmates? This is discussed more in depth later, but is still important to know at the beginning of the process.

Will you survive financially?

If you're anything like me, you don't like discussing money too much and in fact will try to avoid it but in this case, this is a subject that you need to address head on. You will have to honestly ask yourself (and your spouse) if you will survive financially. Why you ask? Because a lot of the time, once your program gets going, the requirements of the program start to take over a majority of your life, leaving less time for work (let alone family and friends). I suggest really talking/thinking about this because working part-time most likely comes with the territory, and if that's something that just isn't an option, then it's good to know now. It doesn't mean that you can't start a program and succeed; it just means that you may have a harder time at it and will have to really organize your schedule. Make sure that if this is you, you figure out great time management, kids, spouse, and life, before you get started and in the thick of things. It will make the program go a lot smoother, with no unexpected conflicts.

How much are you willing to spend/can you afford it?

Sorry to say, but graduate school is not cheap! When I started my program I still had student loans from undergrad that I had been paying off, going in to graduate school. Luckily, that's all I had so I really didn't have much to think about when it came to taking out more student loans for graduate school. But, if you have student loans, a house, a car etc. it may effect how much you want to spend on a program, so if this is you, be sure to really look at cost per credit hour and any other extra costs such as lab fees and simulation bags, because these can add up too. Don't worry though; you're not the only one. And, the good news is, after you graduate, you'll have a job with a bit more income to help pay for all that education!

How will it effect your family and those around you?

The decision to go back to school is a big decision and it's one that you should definitely talk over with your significant other and even your parents, siblings and friends; it will affect everyone around you. You'll have to take out student loans, you'll have to work less which requires you to rely on your significant other or whoever, for extra income or financial support. And honestly, you're going to be hard to deal with emotionally. If you ask anybody's significant other how that person acted during graduate school, hell even just undergrad nursing school, they're going to tell you they were crazy. They're going to tell you that they were stressed out all the time and that they could barely handle them. My husband and I dated when I was completing my undergrad nursing degree so he was witness to the emotional ups and downs, stress and anxiety of undergrad. So, he dreaded me going back to school, knowing what was to come. I calmly stated that this time around things wouldn't be as bad because I was older, more mature, and could handle stress a lot better...boy was I wrong. Graduate School takes a toll on you psychologically, physically and emotionally. When you're in graduate school you realize how much you don't know and it makes you second-guess everything you do and have ever done as a nurse. It makes you wonder how the heck you have kept your patients alive all this time and it makes you question everything you do. For some people this can mess with your emotions and confidence and can make us wonder, "why I am a nurse" or "wow I really don't know anything" when in fact you do, you're just being opened up too a much of broader range of everything. When we are nurses we just have a bubble of information that is specialized to a specific area. But when you go to graduate school that bubble gets popped, and you learn everything. You realize that you only knew just a little bit, of a whole bunch of information. It will humble you and it will overwhelm you, but by the end of your program, hopefully, you will realize that you have learned more than you thought, and will have gained some life long friends along the way. You will say to yourself, "I think I can do it, I think I know this stuff," and you'll gain that confidence back. The confidence will not be there at the beginning of your program, but it will return by the end.

Types of Advanced Practice Nurse Concentrations

Family Nurse Practitioner/Adult Nurse Practitioner (FNP/ANP)- These types of nurse practitioners usually work in primary care/clinics or in the hospital but on medical-surgery floors (some do work in ICUs but I know with the recent consensus model, they're trying to phase these NPs out if the ICU and require an ACNP certification if working in the ICU as an NP). Prerequisites are pretty much the same for every program, and they're all usually obtained within your BSN education so no extra prerequisite education should be required. Education is mostly online and can be completed within 1-2 years; depending on how many classes you want to take in a semester. I have friends that continue to work full time while obtaining their FNP and it usually takes them two years so it's definitely doable.

Clinical Nurse Specialist (CNS)- A CNS is usually associated with quality improvement. What I mean by that? Quality improvement has to do with preforming tasks or actions that can lead to a measurable improvement in patient population. CNSs tend to work in the hospital with service lines, but depending on where you go have been used interchangeably with NPs in the ICU. For example, our CNS in my ICU doesn't do that much patient care, but she does a lot with ST Elevated Myocardial Infarction

(STEMI) protocols and improving the time it takes to get someone to the cardiac catheterization lab when a STEMI is suspected. Like an NP program, prerequisites are the same and a CNS program can take about a year to two, again, depending on the student, program, and the specialty. Like NPs, CNS can specialized in adults, pediatrics, psych/mental health, home health and public health, but there aren't a lot of programs so specific specialty programs may be hard to find.

Acute Care Nurse Practitioner (ACNP)- ACNPs are just starting to be used more. The role was created to help fill in gaps or assist with the management of patients to reduce inpatient load; a lot of times, the ACNP and Physician Assistant roles are used interchangeably. An ACNP typically works in acute care environments (obviously) that include ICUs and Emergency Departments mostly. An ACNP acts as intensivist so their skill set is very different and more involved than the FNP/ANP. An ACNP performs invasive procedures like central line placement, chest tube insertion, intubations and etc. so it can't be done online successfully; it needs to be done in class. Academically, there are no extra prerequisites necessary, however, professionally, most schools do prefer that you have at least a year of ICU experience, sometimes two, depending on the program. Most programs are between 18 and 26 months so they definitely vary in terms of length and content.

Certified Registered Nurse Anesthetist (CRNA)- These are nurses who administer anesthesia under the supervision of an anesthesiologist (although the anesthesiologist is usually never in the room, just the vicinity). Some schools require at least a year of ICU experience, others two. Depending on the program they require prerequisites like organic chemistry and physics (since these aren't usually offered in BSN program you would have to get these separately on your own time). The programs usually take 24-30 months, nonstop and they suggest that you don't work. In some places the job market might be a bit more competitive, so that would be something to consider if you're thinking about taking this route.

Psychiatric-Mental Health Nurse Practitioner (PMHNP)- These NPs are in high demand and tend to work in outpatient community mental health clinics, usually under the supervision of a medical doctor who specializes in psychiatric-mental health. The PMHNP education can be completed online in 18-24months, depending on the pace you go. Just like other APRN specialties, some programs may require that you have some mental health nursing experience or that you have evidence of mental health nursing experience in undergrad. As stated earlier, these NPs are in high demand in just about every region, so the job outlook is very good.

Pediatric Nurse Practitioner (PNP)- These NPs work with neonatal patients, children and adolescents. The PNP tends to work inpatient, outpatient or both. Chances are you can even see them in the Pediatric ICU so depending on the type of program, they may require PICU experience. Undergraduate prerequisites are the same as any other NP specialty, but they do require previous pediatric nursing experience. Program length is 2-3 years with options to choose between on-campus/in-class programs and online programs. These NPs are in high demand as well so the job outlook is positive.

Certified Nurse Midwife (CNM)- These APRNs focus a majority of their care on gynecologic, obstetrics, childbirth and newborn care, but have also been used for primary care needs related to reproductive issues and prevention. These APRNs tend to work in the hospitals, outpatient clinics, private homes and public health clinics. Most CNM programs require the same prerequisites as other APRN programs and can be completed within 12-18 months, with online option available.

Nurse Educator- If you like taking students (if you are a preceptor) and teaching, this may be for you. Usually a nurse educator will be an educator for intensive care units/specific floors, or they are a nursing instructor for undergraduates and graduates. Prerequisites for nurse education may require that you have some preceptor and nursing experience but other than that, all other prerequisites and program length are the same as FNP/ANP/CNS.

Nurse Administrator/Executive/Clinical Nurse Leader- If you're that nurse who likes being in charge and is involved in committees, then this route may be your thing. This route tends to be paper and research heavy (depending on where you go) and can usually take 2 years. People who have this degree tend to hold positions such as nurse manager, all the way to chief nursing officer (although most of the time, you would also have to have your MBA or MHA). Prerequisites for this may require leadership experience such as preceptor or a charge nurse/supervisor.

Nurse Informatics- Nurse informatics is for nurses who like technology, and know how to integrate it into today's practice. These nurses can work for software companies as a consult or a facility itself to help buffer the complications that comes with integrating technology and the daily responsibilities of nursing. Education for this specialty usually takes 2 years part-time and can be done online.

Post-Masters Certificate- These programs are for those who already have a Masters in Nursing, but want to change or broaden their specialties. Typically, these versions of a specialty program are shorter because the candidate doesn't have to complete the core masters nursing courses, just the specialty courses. Just about every specialty offers a post-masters program, some more than others. The only draw back is that there aren't that many out there so it may be difficult to find one that is close to you.

Choosing the Right Program

When considering going to grad school I recommend that you first decide which advanced practice route you want to take and then choose a program by the curriculum that best suits you. I believe it's really important to look at the curriculum of a program you're considering because it may not be the right one for the position that you want to have when you are done. Also, I recommend you sit down and think about what type of student you are. Are you a student that does OK online studying, mostly independently, or are you a student that does better in class. Knowing this will definitely have an effect which program you apply to and your success within the program. I also recommend when researching a program, looking at accreditation, attrition rate, length of the program, and cost, all these factors are going to play into which program will be the best for you to succeed and achieve your goals.

I hate to say this but not all graduate schools/programs are created equal so that's important to keep in mind. When you go to apply for a job after graduation your employer shouldn't have to question where you got your degree from, with that being said... look at the coursework, look at the clinical hours, do they meet the requirements for your field? And, if you're not sure about something do not hesitate to email the coordinator or the director and simply ask them. I'm sure they would welcome the question and your interest in their program. When considering going back to school, take a look at the APRN consensus model. This model was basically designed to provide a clearer definition and differentiation between advanced practice roles. This model has been made and is currently in the process of being implemented into healthcare systems across the US, so some APRN roles may be adjusted.

Online vs. In-Class

There are mainly two types of programs, online and in-class. The advantages one gets from an online program is that most of the time these can be completed while still working full time and at your own pace, with maybe one to two required in-class visits per year. They also allow you to work in your own environment, at a lower cost. These programs are great for people who are self-disciplined, still have to work full time and don't want to have to commute every week. One disadvantage from these, however, is that if you don't understand a concept or management strategy, it may be a bit more difficult to get help. Another disadvantage is that usually, online programs require you to find your own preceptors for clinical so if you're in an area where the closest possible preceptor is miles away or there aren't any very well established, this can be very difficult and cause a lot of stress. The advantages one gets from an in-class program is that you get face-to-face interaction with your instructors, as well as your classmates, and the opportunity to have a more "hands on" experience. This allows you to build relationships and better understand concepts and management, which leads to increased success in the program. Another advantage is that in-class programs tend to already have preceptors picked for clinical, which eliminates that hassle of finding one. Some disadvantages of in-class programs include limited flexibility, higher tuition, and possible distracting environments. The end goal is to obtain your degree so it is important to look at the pros and cons of each type of program, and then figure out which one you would be the most successful at and go for it!

Inpatient vs. Outpatient

Whether you want to be inpatient or outpatient is going to effect the program that you choose, so therefore you should probably determine what kind of environment you want to work in as advanced practice nurse. Do you want to keep working in the hospital or do you want to work in more of an outpatient clinic. There are pros and cons to each environment but the most important thing is that you know which one you want to ultimately work in because it may be very hard to switch in the middle of your program or after. For example most ACNPs/CNSs are inpatient, whereas most FNPs do outpatient. ANPs/CNMs are kind of in the middle where they will do outpatient but you can also see them taking on a hospitalist role within the hospital. When it comes to CRNA jobs there really isn't an issue between inpatient and outpatient because all CRNAs are trained the same and whether you do inpatient anesthesia vs. outpatient anesthesia it's pretty much all the same. The CNS rules mainly in patients and may be outpatient for quality improvement project reasons but they're mainly inpatient.

Class size

This is something that you can consider but it doesn't have to be a deal-breaker. Some schools especially CRNA schools, will only offer sizes of 6 people maximum, whereas other schools would offer sizes as big as 32 people. For applying, ideally the bigger class size would increase the chances of you being admitted, but you have to keep in mind that the bigger the class size the bigger the instructor to student ratio, so success and individualization within the program may be a little bit more difficult than the smaller class sizes.

Prerequisites

When it comes to prerequisites for NP/CNS/CNM school, they're usually all obtained through your undergraduate program so you shouldn't have to take any additional courses. HOWEVER, keep in mind that for some schools, they will only accept your sciences for so many years after they have been completed. In regards to CRNA school, most schools require at least biochemistry, physics, or organic chemistry to be completed either during the submission of your application or before. So preparation for this application process usually starts 6 months-1 year before the actual submission of your application. For both ACNP and CRNA schools, ICU experience is a prerequisite as well. A majority say a minimum of one year but two years preferred. Lastly, look at what certifications the school requires. Some just require Basic Life Support (BLS), while others will want BLS, Advanced Cardiac Life Support (ACLS), Pediatric Advanced Life Support (PALS) and/or your Critical Care Registered Nurse (CCRN) certification. If you don't have these but they're required for application submission, make sure you sign up or study for these ASAP because classes fill up way in advance.

The Application Process

The actual application process is pretty straightforward. Usually it will include an application with a fee, request for transcript (which usually costs $10-$15), request for letters of recommendation, request for a resume or curriculum vitae and an essay. Some schools may have a questionnaire that they would like you to fill out as well, to assess nurse competencies. Some schools may even require one of those lovely personality tests as part of your application. Make sure you submit it at least a week before the deadline, just to make sure everything gets in on time and is accounted for.

Resume/Curriculum Vitae

Most places will ask for one or the other. The difference between the two is that a resume usually consists of your name, contact information, work experience, and education. A curriculum vitae (CV) consists of the same components as the resume but also includes professional achievements and memberships, publications, and references. If you haven't achieved all of the components on the CV, it's ok, just put what you have done so far. I've been told that the CV is a place where you get to brag about your accomplishments and achievements on paper.

Essay/Personal Statement

I know as soon as you see the word essay you groan, there is a reason we went into nursing and not journalism, right? But, if you've gone through your nursing program you've already figured out that we still do quite a bit of writing in school, and it only increases in volume when you go for your Master's or Doctorate. The essay doesn't need to be long, but should not be super short either. For the NP/CNS/CNM student, the personal statement usually consists of where you work, what makes you a good candidate and your career goals. For CRNAs, they usually just want to know why you want to be a CRNA. So, look at the essay as a place to brag on yourself a little bit. Mention your experience with your patient population and how you have grown as a nurse. If you have helped on any committees or research projects, mention that.

Letters of Recommendation

My advice would be to have the forms for each school you are applying to, all together in one envelope and deliver each person their own envelope of recommendation forms. This way, all the letter of recommendations get done at the same time, get sent out at the same time, and decreases the amount of work for the person filling out or writing the letter of recommendation. Don't forget to thank them for helping you out. A thank you card with a nice message is usually a good way to do it.

The Interview Process

The interview process is the process that can determine whether or not you get into a program so being prepared is VITAL to acceptance.

Research the Program

As stated before it is very important that you research the program you interview for. You should know the range of students they accept each year, their attrition rate, and successful job placement percentage. Every program is different so it's important to look at their coursework as well. Looking at a program's coursework allows you to see what the program is about and where they put emphasis. Some programs will have more science and less theory, while others will have more theory with the minimum amount of science. Some programs will have more research, while others will have less. Some will have a year of just didactic before clinical. Some will start clinical from day one all they way through. This will be good to know, just in case you have any questions.

Know Your Specialty

This is a given, but it's always good to be reminded and prepared. During some interviews they will ask you about your skills and how you care for patients in your area of expertise. They're usually common scenarios you would see in your specialty, so they're not meant to be hard. They just want to see if you know how to take care of the basic management, they will teach you how to take it further. I am a cardiac ICU nurse so the question I was asked in my interview was "Your patient just went into atrial fibrillation, what would you do?" Pretty straightforward right? I once had a friend tell me that in her CRNA interview, they gave her the scenario "your mechanically ventilated patient starts to de-sat, what would you do?" This is a pretty general question and obviously, there are a lot if things you can do, but the goal of the question is that they want to assess your thinking process. They're assessing if you have the capability to independently manage a patient (of course while still being within your current scope of practice); that you're thinking.

Know Your Pharmacology

If you are an ICU nurse interviewing for CRNA or ACNP school, you will need to know your vasoactive drugs and which receptors they effect. If you work in a specific specialty such as cardiac or neuroscience, know the most common medications and doses used. In some interviews, they may not ask about specific doses, but it never hurts to be prepared. What really helped me when I interviewed was that, I reviewed the notes that I had taken when I studied to obtain my CCRN certification, however, I realize this may not apply to everyone (especially depending on what type of program you're applying to).

Know Your Strengths and Weaknesses

I believe regardless of the field your interviewing for this question will come up. To prepare for this section of the interview, in regards to your strengths, I would advise you to really sit down and assess yourself. What are you good at? What skills do you have? What makes you, uniquely you? In nursing, some great strengths to have are patience, dedication, flexibility, and being a team player. The trick to answering this question, in regards to your weakness, is to make sure your weakness can be twisted into a positive weakness (but still be honest of course). For example, a positive weakness can be "I don't feel comfortable going to lunch until all my charting is done, and my patient is taken care of (which is true)". This tells them that sure you sometimes have a late lunch and tend to ignore your own health, but it's only because you're concentrating on patient care and documentation, and those are much more important to you than eating. It's not that you don't want them to know the real you, you just want to make sure you're always showing your best, even at your weakest.

Know your Financial Plan

If they ask you about work or financial status once in the program, have a plan. You don't have to know the specifics but just have a general idea of how you're going to pay for school, books, and living expenses (loans vs. scholarship vs. out-of-pocket). This shows them that not only have you planned ahead, but also, that you're already somewhat dedicated to the program and everything it entails. If you are interviewing for a CRNA or ACNP program, don't be surprised if they mention that they prefer students to work part-time or not at all. These programs are very intense and require a lot of dedication to your studies so you will rarely have time for a personal life, let alone work.

Prepare to Share Your Goals and Achievements

Some committees will ask you what you have achieved both in the nursing community and your personal community. This is the chance for you to brag about yourself so go for it! Grad schools want the best of the best. They want the nurses who go above and beyond. They want the nurses that volunteer in soup kitchens three nights a week, hold positions on councils at work, raise the kids, keep the house clean, and have dinner on the table by six (okay, a little exaggerated but you get the idea). Also, be prepared to share your long-term goals. What area do you want to work in once you graduate? Where would you like to go/where do you see yourself in five years? How will this program help you achieve that goal? They just want to know you and how you intend on using your degree once graduated.

Be Up to Date on What is Happening in the Advanced Practice World

Some schools like their students to be active and engaged in the advanced practice nurse community so they may ask you about/or to name a current event in nursing that could affect your future practice, positive or negative. How do you prepare for this? Read some recent articles and/or studies. Where can you find some? Everywhere. Go to your state board of nursing's website and look at the hot topics being discussed. Some of the big national topics include the implementation of the consensus model, the push for a universal scope of practice across all 50 states, and prescriptive authority. Having this knowledge will show the committee that you are already concerned and vested in the APRN career.

Be Prepared to Talk About Unrelated Nursing Topics

I've had people tell me that in their interviews, they were not asked any clinical questions, but rather personal questions such as, "what was the last book or research article you have read." One question I have been asked is "tell me something about you that your resume doesn't tell me?" These are tough questions because we don't expect them to ask anything about us personally (unrelated to their program), so when they do, we blank. We aren't prepared to talk about something so simple, ourselves. Ultimately, what it comes down to is that they want to get to know you, what kind of student you are, and if you're right for their program. If there are some bad grades on your transcript, be prepared to explain why it happened and don't be afraid to be honest. If your grades dipped due to too much partying, tell them that, but follow up with the fact that you've matured since then. I am all about being honest and open in an interview because nothing good comes from dishonesty. Eventually, they will find out.

What to do Next?

You've turned in your application, had your interview and now, you play the waiting game, until you become Person A or Person B.

Person A: Congratulations, you got into graduate school! Now for the next 2 years you'll be busy studying, writing, rounding and more. It would probably be best to sit down with your family and figure out a game plan for the upcoming year.

Finances

As far as finances go, if you plan on obtaining a federal loan, fill out your FAFSA as soon as you can. If your interested in scholarships, email your school to see if you qualify for any, or go online and find an association that is related to the field you want to go into. Different associations offer different types of scholarships for both undergraduate and graduate students when they plan to pursue a certain specialty of nursing. It may not be enough to cover all of your tuition, but every little bit can help.

Work

This may be hard to do at this moment, but try to assess whether you can actually go to working part-time or not. This is a conversation that needs to occur as well because it's very different talking about it, than actually going through with it.

Relax

Relax and enjoy what time you have now because you may not get to play your computer games or do your outdoor activities that often for the next 2 years. If you can, take a vacation and enjoy some time with your loved ones. I'm not saying you absolutely won't have time to do these things, I'm just saying that once you start graduate school and get a chance to relax or take a vacation, you're going to have what you should actually be doing for school running in the back of your mind, hindering any enjoyment that you could have.

Person B: So you went through the application process, the interview process, and played the waiting game, but you didn't get in. Don't feel bad it happens more often than you know. It actually happened to me two years in a row. Don't let it effect you, it does not mean you are an incompetent nurse; it only means that you just weren't what they were looking for this year. So how can you strengthen your application so you will get in the next time?

Ask About Your Application

One thing I did the second time I was rejected was that I

emailed the director or the program coordinator. First of all, I wanted to thank them for considering me for an interview and then asked them how I could strengthen my application so I could be a better candidate for the next year. I have found that a lot of times they will tell you that they would like more experience, certifications, or in a CRNA school situation, evidence of biochemistry or physics classes. I encourage you to do this the first time, and not be afraid to ask. Just like when you researched the program, they will welcome your desire for feedback. This will show them that you're really interested in their program and want to become the best candidate possible.

Continue Education

A lot of the time, they question why you don't have a certain certification specific to your specialty and they suggest that you probably get it for the next round of applications to be a better candidate. If you are in the ICU, obtaining your CCRN would be the way to go. If you are in a trauma unit or in the ED, your Trauma Nursing Core Course (TNCC) certification would be something good to have as well. Having these certifications by all means DOES NOT mean that one nurse's abilities are better than the other's, it just shows the committee that you're very interested in continuing your education and are willing to put in the extra time and effort, outside of work.

Look at Your Letters of Recommendation

Take a second and look at your recommendations. Did you choose the supervisor that is your best friend and then some other random person that you happen to work well with? Perhaps next time, choose people that are high up in the career ladder like your nurse manager or one of the attending physicians that you work with. It's not that your best friend the supervisor wouldn't give you a good recommendation, it's just that sometimes, they're not the most professional. Selecting committees want to see that you are highly recommended so they really like to see candidates that have high profile health care professionals such as physicians as references. When a physician recommends you, this tells them that the physician trusts you with their patients and believes that you are a competent nurse, which in turn can say a lot about you and your nursing abilities.

Look at your Experience

Sometimes the only thing holding you back is experience. If that is the case, there's really nothing more you can do other than, gain more experience. How can you do this? The obvious one would be to continue working until the next application deadline comes around, but perhaps change up your patient assignments. If you don't get the sick patients that often, ask to take them. The great thing about the nursing profession is that you're always learning, so no matter how much experience you have, you can always gain more. However, if you feel like you've learned everything you can in your unit, start picking up shifts on other floors or in other ICUs, this will greatly expand your education and make you knowledgeable of more than one specialty, which can help you look that much better to a admissions committee when you reapply.

www.ingramcontent.com/pod-product-compliance
Lightning Source LLC
Chambersburg PA
CBHW071833200526
45169CB00018B/1418